I0146752

Mastering

the

Sway Test

By: Brenda Anderson

Copyright © by Brenda Anderson
Little Lost Creations

Revised 2019
All rights reserved. This book or any portion thereof may not be
reproduced or used in any manner whatsoever without the
express written permission of the publisher.

www.littlelostcreations.net

Use at your own discretion not to take the place of
medical advice.

Dedicated to everyone that has taught me in one way or another and helped me learn.

I am grateful for all of the herbs, oils, ect.. and everything I have learned. This knowledge, along with blessings from our Heavenly Father, have helped me heal my body while going through a serious illness.

Sometimes we have to go through these trials of Faith to force us to move out of our comfort zone and take control of our lives.

Muscle Testing

Mastering the Sway Test

When I learned how to muscle test I thought I was signed up for an essential oils class. I had never really learned much about Kinesiology or what some people call muscle testing. When the class started the teacher had us stand up to learn muscle testing using the sway test. My first thought was, I am in the wrong class!

After a few minutes in the class I rememberer thinking I will never learn how to do this. After 4 days of class I left determined I could master muscle testing if I just concentrate and work at it. So I went home and practiced for an entire month before the next series of classes. This was in 2004.

I did learn how to test and now I teach classes to others. Since then I have learned many other interesting modalities, and other natural options such as oils, tinctures, homeopathic. Muscle testing helps me know what to use and how to use it.

I enjoy the skills I have learned and use them on a daily basis to test and help myself, family and friends.

For those of you who don't know what muscle testing is, let me explain my version of it. We all have an energy system. Let me explain briefly about our energy system. This can be very complex and takes a lot more in depth study, this is my short version.

When I first started to learn about muscle testing and our energy system I thought this is crazy. These words sound scary and didn't really make sense to me. After I learned they are Chinese words I started to understand. In our English language we don't have a word for Aura, Meridian,

Chakra's and others, so the Chinese words are used.

Our Energy System

Now we have our physical bodies that we see and feel. We can actually feel how much physical energy we have. Our bodies also have a vital energy which is the energy we use to operate our heart, brain and other organs.

Around our physical bodies we have many energy layers which is called an Aura. Each of these layers are a different color varying from person to person. They each give off a vibrating energy.

Chakras

We also have 7 Chakras on our bodies that are like an electrical substation or a power plant. These chakras are down the middle of our body starting at the tailbone. This chakra is called a Root chakra. The Root Chakra is numbered as one and they move up the body towards the head. The number seven chakra is the Crown Chakra on the top of the head. There are many more chakras that surround our bodies, but I am going to try to keep this simple. Each of these chakra's spin in the opposite direction of each other and works as an energy station.

Meridians

A meridian is like a power line that runs through our organs and through our chakras. While passing through our chakra a meridian picks up energy and takes it along the

meridian path carrying the energy to our organs.

This is a crash course, simplified version of how I view aura's, chakra's and meridians.

I try to keep it simple so even a beginner can understand how the energy system works.

Feeling Energy

What do you think energy feels like?

We can learn how to feel the energy in our bodies and also the energy around us. I feel that through muscle testing we can use our subconscious mind, and or spirit to communicate and find out what our body needs emotionally, mentally, spiritually and physically to help it heal and stay healthy.

Muscle testing could also be considered intuition. I feel muscle testing is a gift or a talent from God and should be used properly at all times for good.

In this book I will teach you the beginning steps of muscle testing. Once you learn this I will have follow up books to teach other testing techniques and different ways you can use this skill.

There are several things you have to remember about muscle testing. The first

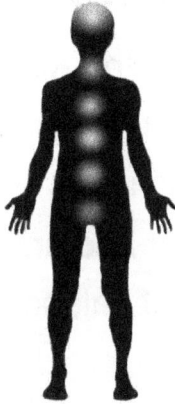

thing you need to do is prepare yourself. It is important to have your body in balance to test. If you are not in balance you will get goofy answers or lots of no's or yeses or you may get no answers at all.

So what does it mean to be in balance? To me it means that I am focused on what I am doing, I am present. My mind, body and soul are in balance and are all working together.

Here are some ways you can get your body in balance

- First your body needs to be well hydrated in order to muscle test. Your body requires the water to help the electrical impulses of energy move through it. So if you are thirsty get a big drink of water and any time you may test you are out of balance start with a drink of water.

- Make sure you are comfortable.

- You can also get into balance by walking on the grass, or rubbing your bare feet in the grass.

- Another way to get into balance is to extend your arms out in front of you, lock your hands together and point your pointer fingers straight out together. Now with your eyes follow your pointer fingers as you do a big figure 8 laying on its side so it is crossing over both sides of your body. This is using both sides of your brain.

* Brain Gym exercises also help.

* Another way is to march in place. Now tap your knee with the palm of your opposite hand left to right, right to left while marching. This is another way of using both sides of your brain to get you into balance.

* Hug a tree. I know this sounds a little crazy but the tree is grounded by its roots that run deep into the ground. Hold onto a branch, touch the trunk or literally hug the tree.

There are many other ways to get grounded and into balance. This is a good list to get you started.

Let's get started

I ask the question a little bit ago "What does energy feel like?" You tell me what does energy feel like?

Energy may not feel the same to everyone. To some they may feel heat, others may feel tingling or other sensations. What does energy feel like to you? Let's find out.

The first thing I would like you to do is put the palms of your hands together and rub them quickly. What do you feel? Do you feel heat? Do you feel tingling? Whatever you feel, this is what energy feels like to you.

Now that you know what energy feels like let's have a little bit of fun. We are going to make an energy ball.

Rub the palm of your hands together quickly until you can feel the energy. Keep your hands with your palms facing each other, fingers extended, move your hands apart very slowly. Move them slightly in and out. Can you feel a resistance? Can you feel the energy ball. Now move them apart a little farther. How far apart can you get your hands until you no longer feel the energy?

Energy can be found all around us. Let's try gathering some energy and adding it to your energy ball.

Make your energy ball once again. Cup your hand slightly and move it outwards and then back in like you are gathering something and adding to a ball. Can you feel the energy? Now do the opposite hand. Move inwards until you feel resistance like you are holding the ball. Cup your hand, move it out like you are gathering more energy and adding it to the ball. Can you feel the ball growing? Keep repeating these steps until your ball gets the size you want it.

Mastering the Sway Test

Now we are going to work with your energy system in a different way. You use your energy while muscle testing. There are many ways to muscle test, but I am going to teach you the sway test in this book. I teach this technique because it is the easiest for you to start with and the easiest to feel.

What is the sway test? The sway test is a way that we can communicate with our energy systems. Our bodies naturally move forward to things that are good for us and move away from things that are not good for us. When we talk to our bodies they naturally move towards things that are good for us.

The language we use when talking to our bodies is very important. It is important to remember to make statements. The way we word our statements can at times determine the outcome.

You will notice that I tell you to make a statement. It is important to make a statement and not ask a question. Our bodies can only answer a yes or no statement. The body cannot answer a question, so evaluate what you are saying and make sure you are making a statement.

I like to use the word beneficial. (Example) "This oil would be beneficial for me to use."

Notes:

Are you ready to learn the sway test?

1. The first thing you need to do is clear your mind. It is important you clear your mind and do not look at anyone else, especially if you are testing for another person. *(yes testing for someone else can be done and we will learn it a later book)*

2. Now stand up straight planting your feet flat on the ground just a little ways apart. As you sway this will help you keep your balance.

3. I know that this next part may feel a little weird, but as you learn, you will understand talking to your body. Say out loud to your body. **"Body sway forward for yes. Body sway backwards for no."** It is necessary for you to say this out loud to your body so it knows what is expected of it.

4. Now say: **"Show me a yes."** Your body should rock forward. Relax and give your body time to work. If you need to, close your eyes and see if you can feel your body move forward. If you don't feel it sway forward we will work on that in a few minutes.

5. Now say: **"Show me a no."** Your body should rock backwards. Relax and give your body time to work. This is something totally new to your body so it needs to think about it. Again close your eyes and see if you can feel your body move. If you don't feel it, don't worry, you will.

If you felt your body really sway - Great Job!!

If your body is moving opposite of what it should be; backwards for yes and forward for no don't get worried. Just talk with your body and tell it what you expect it to do and which way you want your body to sway. This can be changed easily. At least your body is responding to the sway.

Sometimes it takes a little time to get the hang of this, you will, don't worry. If you could barely feel your body move or if you didn't feel it lets try it again. But first you need to tell your body this statement:

- **Body rock forward really hard for yes!**

- **Body rock backward really hard for no!**

Now go back to steps #3 and #4 and do them again.

Did it work? If so great!! If not take a break and get a drink of water and relax for a minute and do what you need to do, so you can get your body into balance.

Whether you are coming back and trying all of this again or everything worked the first time, I want you to make this statement. This is to test to see if you are in balance.

State: **I am in balance.**

Did you feel yourself sway forward or backwards? If you went forward, great! If you went backwards go back to the section where we talk about balancing your body. Do at least one of those exercises. When you have completed it then make the statement again. **"I am in balance."**

"I am in balance" is a statement you make each time you start to muscle test. If you are not in balance do one fo the exercises to balance your body.

Now if you were having trouble feeling the sway it is time to talk to your body again. Tell your body what you are expecting of it. It is important to talk to your body. I know that it feels a little strange but just work at it, you will get used to it. You will be talking to it a lot even after you master the sway test. Tell your body... **"body, this is what I need you to do. I need you to rock hard forward for a yes and rock hard backwards for a no."**

Now it is time to test

- **Body show me a yes.**

- **Body show me a no.**

I am sure you could feel it now. If not take another break and then come back and try again. Sometimes it is hard to feel yourself move. You may be moving just a little bit but not actually feeling it. If this is the case have someone stand watching the side of you to see if you are actually moving, and moving in the right direction. Continue practicing this until you can feel your body sway.

There is no rush, relax, take your time and believe it will work.

When you can feel your body swaying forward for yes and backwards for no you have accomplished it. **You** can muscle test using the sway! Now that you can test, what are you going to use it for?

This is your assignment. Start testing everything you can find to test.

I would like you to go around your kitchen and gather up things that you can practice with. An apple, a bottle of vitamins, essential oils, anything you can find to test, even junk food. Go to the grocery store and test foods you are going to buy. Go to the health food store and test vitamins and supplements on the shelf. Have some fun with what you are doing. The more you practice the more you will learn, and you will become proficient at muscle testing.

Setting up statements

The next step is to learn your wording for testing something.

I like to use the word **beneficial**. The word beneficial means this would be good for my body to eat or use.

I try to stay away from using the word need. You may need 8 glasses of water, but is it beneficial for you to drink 8 glasses of water at once? It probably wouldn't be good for you all at once. That is why I like to use the word beneficial.

In the next ebooks you will learn more about wording and why you would use the word beneficial. I think it is easier to start out with good wording so you don't have to try and break a bad habit.

This is what I would say:
"It is beneficial for me to ...."

Now you are going to get some funny answers to some of the things you test. Say for instance you test an apple. Now you know that an apple is good for you unless you are allergic to it. So you would say; "This apple is beneficial for me to eat." Say you get a no.

You would think this apple is good for you but why would it test no? I would then ask.

This apple is beneficial for me to eat if I peel it. Now you get a yes? Maybe there is a wax or a chemical in the peeling that would not be good for you to eat. Interesting huh!

Bottled water is another fun one to play with. You would think the expensive bottles of water would be the best for you. This is not always the case when you test them. If you get a no on a bottle of water test to see if you poured the water into a glass container, would it be beneficial for you. If you still get a no it is probably not the greatest water for you to drink.

Sometimes it is the plastic bottle that the water is in that isn't testing good, and sometimes it is the water itself.

Let's say you test a can of green beans. You and a friend are testing together. Using the same can of green beans, you test the can of green beans are not beneficial for you, but your friend gets they are beneficial.

Look at your diets. Maybe they are not beneficial for you because you are a healthy eater and your body is used to fresh beans or eating something better. Now the person testing with you gets the can of green beans is beneficial for them. Maybe they are not a healthy eater and a can of green beans is better than no green beans.

Remember when testing we are not all the same. What tests good for you may not test good for someone else.

These are just a few examples of how you can practice your muscle testing. The main thing you need to remember is the wording. Always make a statement and use the word beneficial. You also need to remember to practice, practice, practice and it will come to you.

This book is just a start for muscle testing. In the next book I will teach different techniques, you can use, besides the sway test. I will also teach you other things you can test for. Muscle testing is a great way for you to figure out what is going on with your body. If you are sick, muscle testing can help you determine what you can do to help heal your body.

Once you can feel the sway when you test, continue practicing until you feel confident. When you feel confident you are ready to move to the next book.

Please go back to Little Lost Creations or Amazon and give this book a review. I hope you enjoyed it.

If you are looking for more interesting things to read go to my blogs at:

https://littlelostcreations.net

and https://brendaskidsbooks.com

Thank you for purchasing my book!

Happy Testing!

(Tip)When I take a class I always write my notes in my books. I found if I write notes on papers or notebooks they get misplaced. I can always find them in my books.

Notes:

www.ingramcontent.com/pod-product-compliance
Lightning Source LLC
Chambersburg PA
CBHW062122040426
42336CB00041B/2234